The Right Trauma Therapy for You

EMDR, Brainspotting, and Deep Brain Reorienting Explained and Compared

How Each One Works, Who It Helps, and How to Choose with Confidence

Rudolph Alfred Boyd

This book is published for educational and informational purposes only. It is not medical advice, psychological treatment, or a substitute for care from a qualified professional. The author and publisher are not providing therapy through these pages, and reading this book does not create a clinician and client relationship. Decisions about trauma treatment should always be made together with a licensed mental health professional or physician who knows your history. If you are in crisis or experiencing thoughts of harming yourself, contact your local emergency services or a crisis line in your region before doing anything else.

All named individuals appearing in case examples in this book are fictional composites created to illustrate common patterns. They do not describe real clients, and any resemblance to actual persons, living or dead, is coincidental. Descriptions of therapy sessions are illustrative and simplified, and real sessions will differ.

The author and publisher make no warranties, express or implied, about the completeness or accuracy of the information in this book, and disclaim all liability for any loss, injury, or damage allegedly arising from its use. Research on the therapies described here continues to develop, and findings summarized in these pages may be refined or revised by later studies. The reader assumes full responsibility for how this information is used.

EMDR, Brainspotting, and Deep Brain Reorienting are the names of therapeutic approaches associated with their respective developers and training organizations. This book is an independent publication and is not affiliated with, endorsed by, or sponsored by any of those organizations.

First edition: 2026.
ISBN: 979-8-90599-844-7
Staten House

Table of Contents

Preface

Research on trauma treatment has advanced considerably over the past three decades, and public understanding has advanced with it. Most readers now accept that traumatic experience is held in the body as well as in memory, and that conversation alone does not always reach it. What has not kept pace is guidance on choosing between the treatments this understanding produced. A person who accepts that they need bottom-up therapy still faces three serious options with similar promises, incompatible explanations, and almost no neutral literature comparing them.

Those options are EMDR, Brainspotting, and Deep Brain Reorienting. Each works below the level of deliberate thought, using attention, eye position, and bodily awareness to reach material that ordinary conversation passes over. They differ in what they target. EMDR processes specific memories through alternating left and right stimulation. Brainspotting holds a fixed eye position and follows the body's own processing with minimal direction. Deep Brain Reorienting addresses the brainstem-level shock occurring in the first fractions of a second, before emotion arrives. These are not variations on one technique. They rest on different accounts of where the injury is stored.

The gap this book fills is a practical one. Readers researching these treatments encounter material written almost entirely by the developers of individual methods, supplemented by clinic articles produced to attract clients. Both are useful and neither is neutral. The result is that most people select a trauma therapy according to which practitioner is nearest or which method a friend recommends, then interpret a poor match as personal failure. Treatment nonresponse is common enough across all trauma therapies that this interpretation is usually wrong, and it is expensive in time, money, and hope.

This book applies a single principle across all three methods: examine the match between person and treatment before assigning fault to either. Each therapy receives two chapters, one describing the experience of a session and one weighing its evidence honestly, using identical standards throughout. A comparison across nine practical dimensions follows, then a five-factor matching framework covering trauma type, response pattern, material accessibility, processing preference, and practical availability. The intended outcome is specific: a ranked shortlist, a vetted practitioner, and a defensible reason for the choice.

The primary readers are adults considering or continuing trauma treatment, particularly those whose previous therapy produced understanding without sufficient relief. Counseling students and early-career clinicians deciding which modality training to pursue will find the same comparative material useful for a different purpose, as will practitioners wanting a clear account of approaches outside their own training.

What follows is not a treatment manual, and it contains no protocols for processing traumatic material without professional support. These therapies are relational by design, and the session descriptions here serve preparation and selection rather than self-application. Nor does the book name a superior method, because the evidence does not support one and the question itself is poorly formed. Findings summarized here will develop further, particularly for the newest of the three approaches. What this book offers is the information needed to choose well among three legitimate options, and to recognize when a choice needs revising.

Introduction

You have probably done more work on yourself than most people you know. Morag certainly had. Eleven years of therapy, on and off, with four different practitioners. She could describe her attachment pattern in one sentence and her family system in two. She had a shelf of books with cracked spines and margins full of pencil. And on a Tuesday in March, when a colleague raised his voice in a meeting, her heart slammed against her ribs, her hearing went distant, and she spent the afternoon in the stairwell trying to breathe. That night she typed a question into a search bar: why is therapy not working for me.

If you have typed some version of that question, this book was written for you. Not because something is wrong with you, but because something may be wrong with the match between you and the methods you have tried. Those are different problems, and they have different solutions.

Here is the number that reframes everything. Across studies of trauma-focused psychotherapy, a large share of people do not respond sufficiently to the treatment they receive, with reviews reporting nonresponse in a substantial minority and sometimes approaching half of participants, alongside meaningful dropout rates (Schottenbauer et al., 2008; Lewis, Roberts, Andrew, et al., 2020; Lewis, Roberts, Gibson, & Bisson, 2020). Read that carefully. These are good therapies, delivered in research settings by trained clinicians, and still a large group walks away without enough relief. If effort and honesty were all it took, those numbers would look very different.

Fit Before Fault

This book runs on one principle, and I want to name it before anything else. I call it Fit Before Fault: when a legitimate therapy fails to help a committed person, examine the fit between method and person before assigning fault to either one. Not every method reaches every kind of trauma, and not every nervous system tolerates every kind of processing. A mismatch is not a moral event. It is an engineering problem, and engineering problems can be worked.

Fit Before Fault changes how you read your own history. The therapy that stalled stops being evidence that you are beyond help and becomes a data point about what your system needs. It also changes how you choose what comes next. Instead of asking which therapy has the best reputation, you ask which therapy is built for the specific shape of your difficulty. That question has real answers, and this book will help you find yours.

What This Book Compares

Three therapies sit at the center of these pages. EMDR, which stands for Eye Movement Desensitization and Reprocessing, is the oldest and most researched of the three, endorsed by major clinical guidelines around the world. Brainspotting grew out of EMDR in the early 2000s and works through a fixed eye position rather than moving ones, with the body leading more of the process. Deep Brain Reorienting, usually shortened to DBR, is the newest arrival, developed by a psychiatrist in Scotland and aimed at the brainstem-level shock that occurs in the first instants of a traumatic event.

Why these three and not the dozens of other trauma treatments? Because they form a family. Each one claims to reach below ordinary conversation, into the parts of the brain where trauma responses live. Each one was created or shaped by clinicians who watched talk-based methods stall. And each one is the answer someone will eventually suggest to you if your search continues. Understanding them as a family, with a shared inheritance and real differences, is the fastest way to understand your options.

Other respected approaches exist, including somatic experiencing, sensorimotor psychotherapy, and trauma-focused cognitive therapies. You will see them mentioned where they matter. They are simply not the subject of this comparison, and pretending to compare everything is the surest way to compare nothing well.

What You Will Be Able to Do

By the final chapter, you will be able to do five things you likely cannot do today. You will be able to explain, in plain language, why insight alone did not settle your body. You will be able to describe what actually happens in an EMDR session, a Brainspotting session, and a DBR session, and what each method assumes about how healing works. You will be able to read the research on all three without being fooled by hype or by cynicism. You will be able to score each method against your own history, symptoms, and preferences using a structured framework. And you will be able to find, question, and choose a practitioner with the confidence of someone who knows exactly what they are looking for.

One promise about tone. Nothing here will talk down to you, and nothing here will drown you in jargon to seem impressive. Where a technical term earns its place, I will define it once, clearly, and keep using plain words around it. Trauma has already cost you enough. A book about healing from it should not cost you a dictionary.

What This Book Asks of You

I ask three things. First, read with a pen. There are moments in nearly every chapter where you will be asked to write something short about your own experience, and those small pieces of writing become the raw material for your decision in Chapter 10. Second, hold your conclusions loosely until the comparison is complete. Many readers arrive with a favorite already in mind, usually the one a friend swears by, and the framework works better when every option gets a fair hearing. Third, involve a professional. This book will make you an informed chooser, and an informed chooser still chooses best in conversation with a qualified clinician who knows their history.

> **Action Challenge:** *Before you turn to Chapter 1, write one sentence that describes what you have tried and where it stalled. Morag's read: I understand my past completely and my body still reacts like it is happening now. Keep your sentence somewhere you can find it. It is the first entry in the file you will build across this book, and by Chapter 10 it will sit at the top of a completed decision.*

The Promise of This Book

Here is where we are going. You are not being handed a verdict, because a verdict about the best trauma therapy would be false the moment it was printed. You are being handed something better: a working knowledge of three serious methods, an honest account of what each can and cannot yet claim, and a framework that turns your own history into the deciding vote. Fit Before Fault, from here to the last page. Turn to Chapter 1 and we will start where every mismatch starts, in the gap between what you know and what your body remembers.

Chapter 1: Why Insight Was Never Enough

Lorcan is mid-sentence when it happens. He is at his kitchen table on a video call, calm, articulate, describing last week's progress to his therapist. Then a door slams two floors down. His shoulders climb toward his ears before the sound has finished echoing. His chest locks. His eyes fix on a point just left of the camera, and for four or five seconds he is not in the conversation at all. When he comes back he laughs, embarrassed, and says the thing he has said a hundred times. I know exactly where this comes from. Knowing has never once stopped it.

Sit with the strangeness of that. A grown man who can trace his startle response to its origin with the precision of a historian, and the tracing changes nothing about the response itself. If understanding were the active ingredient in healing, Lorcan would have been done years ago. So either he is doing understanding wrong, which is what he privately believes, or understanding was never the active ingredient for this kind of problem. This chapter makes the case for the second answer, because the second answer happens to be what the science supports, and because everything else in this book depends on it.

The House With Two Floors

Think of your brain as a house with two floors. The upper floor handles language, analysis, planning, and story. It is where insight lives, where therapy conversations happen, and where you assembled every explanation you have about your past. The lower floor handles survival. It watches for threat, launches the body into readiness, and does its work in fractions of a second, long before the upper floor has finished forming a sentence. Neuroscientists describe these as cortical and subcortical systems, and the critical fact about them is the direction of traffic. In moments of perceived danger, the lower floor does not wait for permission from the upper floor. It acts, and the upper floor finds out afterward (LeDoux, 1996).

Therapies that work through conversation are sometimes called top-down approaches, because they start on the upper floor and hope the benefits travel downward. Often they do. For grief, for relationship patterns, for the meaning we make of our lives, talking helps enormously, and nothing in this book argues otherwise. But trauma responses are lower-floor events. The slammed door reaches Lorcan's survival circuitry directly, and that circuitry fires on its own schedule. This is why a growing family of treatments works bottom-up instead, starting with the body and the fast subcortical systems and letting change climb toward the story (Ogden et al., 2006; van der Kolk, 2014).

I call this the Basement Rule, and it is the named principle of this chapter: trauma is stored below the floor that insight can reach, so lasting change has to happen at the level where the response actually lives. The Basement Rule does not say insight is worthless. It says insight is upstairs, and the alarm system is in the basement, and you cannot rewire a basement by redecorating the living room.

What Trauma Does to Memory

Ordinary memory is a story. It has a beginning, an end, and a time stamp that files it firmly in the past. When you recall it, you know you are recalling. Traumatic memory often fails to file this way. Under extreme stress, the systems that would normally stamp and shelve the experience are disrupted, and fragments of it remain live: sensations, images, body states, and reflexes that carry no time stamp at all. When something in the present resembles the fragment, the body responds as if the original event were happening now, because as far as the basement is concerned, it is (van der Kolk, 2014; Kearney & Lanius, 2022).

This is why Lorcan's response feels so unreasonable to him. His upper floor has a complete, well-ordered account of the past. His lower floor holds an unfiled fragment that a slamming door can activate in under a second. Two floors, two kinds of memory, and only one of them responds to explanation. The therapies in this book differ in many ways, but they share one ambition: to reach the unfiled material and let the nervous system finally complete and file it. Where they differ is in how far down they reach and by what doorway, and those differences will matter a great deal when you choose.

The Window You Work Inside

There is a second piece of shared ground, and it explains why trauma work can fail even when the method is sound. Clinicians describe a window of tolerance, a middle band of activation where you are alert enough to engage with difficult material and settled enough to stay present with it (Siegel, 1999). Above the window is hyperarousal: panic, flooding, rage, the feeling of being swept away. Below it is hypoarousal: numbness, fog, distance, the feeling of being switched off. Meaningful processing happens inside the window. Outside it, in either direction, the experience may be intense but the nervous system is not integrating anything.

Windows vary enormously between people, and trauma tends to narrow them. Someone with a wide window can revisit hard material for long stretches. Someone with a narrow window may tip into flooding or shutdown within minutes, through no lack of courage. This single variable explains a large share of the stories you will hear about therapy going wrong, and it will become one of the five deciding factors in your framework later. A method that respects your window feels challenging but workable. A method that repeatedly throws you outside it feels like drowning, whatever its reputation.

> **Action Challenge:** *For the next three days, practice observation without changing anything. Two or three times a day, ask where you are relative to your own window. Inside it, above it in revved-up activation, or below it in flatness and fog. Keep a small tally. You are gathering baseline data about your nervous system, and that data will vote in Chapter 10.*

When Shutdown Is Protection

Some readers will have noticed that their difficulty rarely looks like panic. It looks like absence. The meeting gets tense and they go somewhere behind their own eyes. This is dissociation, and it deserves a plain description because it is one of the most misunderstood responses in all of mental health. Dissociation is a protective maneuver. When escape is impossible and activation is unbearable, the nervous system can disconnect: from the body, from emotion, from the room (Porges, 2011). In the moment of original danger, this is a mercy. Repeated afterward, it becomes a pattern that makes ordinary life feel muffled and makes some forms of therapy genuinely difficult.

Research has recognized this clearly enough that a dissociative subtype of post-traumatic stress is now formally described, marked by exactly this shift into numbing and disconnection rather than classic fear responses (Lanius et al., 2010). The practical point for this book is simple and consequential. Methods differ in how well they accommodate a person who leaves rather than floods. Some protocols assume you can stay actively engaged with a target memory; a person who dissociates may need extended preparation, a modified approach, or a method built with disconnection in mind from the start. When we compare the three therapies, dissociation will get its own line, because for a large group of readers it is the line that decides.

Why Words Stop at the Stairs

Pull the threads together and Lorcan's mystery dissolves. His trauma response lives in fast subcortical circuitry that acts before language arrives. The material driving it never got filed as past, so present-day echoes reactivate it whole. When activation spikes, he leaves his window of tolerance, and outside the window nothing new can be learned. Every talking session he ever attended happened upstairs, in daylight, in language. The basement never heard a word of it.

None of this means his years of therapy were wasted. Insight built the map he will need for whatever comes next, and a person who understands their history makes a far better partner to any of the three therapies ahead. The Basement Rule simply says the map is not the territory. Something still has to go downstairs. The rest of this book is about the three methods that claim they can, and about how to judge which staircase fits the house you actually live in.

> **Action Challenge:** *Take ten minutes with a notebook and write two short descriptions. First, a moment when understanding genuinely changed something for you. Second, a moment like Lorcan's, when understanding was present and powerless. Label the first upstairs and the second basement. You now have a personal, concrete grip on the distinction this whole field is built around, and you will use both notes when you score the therapies against your own history.*

The Short Version

Insight lives on the upper floor of the brain and trauma lives below it, in survival circuitry that acts faster than language and stores experience without a time stamp. Change has to happen where the response lives, inside a window of tolerance that varies from person to person, with special care for the nervous systems that protect themselves by disconnecting. That is the Basement Rule, and it is the ground all three therapies in this book stand on. What separates them is lineage and method, and lineage is where we go next: one walk in a park in 1987, one trembling eye in 2003, and one Scottish psychiatrist deciding the field had not yet gone deep enough.

Chapter 2: One Family, Three Therapies

In the spring of 1987, a psychologist named Francine Shapiro took a walk through a park, preoccupied by some troubling thoughts. She noticed something odd. As her eyes moved spontaneously back and forth, the thoughts seemed to lose their charge. Most people would have shrugged and walked on. Shapiro built a career on the observation, testing it, formalizing it, and developing it into a structured therapy she called Eye Movement Desensitization and Reprocessing (Shapiro, 2018). Within a decade it had clinical trials behind it. Within two, it appeared in international treatment guidelines. An entire branch of trauma treatment traces back to that walk.

Origin stories like this one matter for a practical reason, not a sentimental one. Every therapy inherits the assumptions of the moment it was born in, the problems its founder was staring at, and the tools that happened to be available. If you know where a method came from, you can predict what it will be good at and where it will strain, often before you read a single study. That is the named principle of this chapter, and I call it the Inheritance Test: to understand any therapy, ask what problem it was invented to solve, because it will always solve that problem best.

This chapter draws the family tree. Three methods, one lineage, and a set of inherited assumptions that will do more to guide your choice than any advertisement ever will.

A Walk Becomes a Protocol

Shapiro's insight might have stayed a curiosity if she had not done something unusual for the era: she standardized it. EMDR grew into an eight-phase protocol with a defined sequence, from history-taking and preparation through the famous eye movements to a closing body scan. The client holds a specific troubling memory in mind while tracking the therapist's fingers, or alternating taps or tones, and the memory is worked until its disturbance drops and a more adaptive belief takes hold. The structure is the point. EMDR was born in a scientific culture that demanded testable procedures, and its founder wanted results that could be measured, replicated, and defended.

Apply the Inheritance Test and the profile appears immediately. EMDR was built around identifiable memories that a person can name, hold, and rate. Its natural home is trauma with a clear address: the crash, the assault, the disaster, the moment everything changed. Its structure made it researchable, which is why it now carries the largest evidence base of the three and the endorsements that come with it (Bisson et al., 2013; World Health Organization, 2013). And the same inheritance predicts its strains, which Chapter 4 will examine honestly: material with no clear memory address, and nervous systems for whom holding a trauma in steady focus is itself overwhelming.

The Slow Wobble

Sixteen years later, in 2003, a therapist named David Grand was conducting a session using a slowed-down variant of EMDR he had developed. As he tracked a client's eyes across her visual field, something interrupted the smooth pursuit. Her eyes wobbled and then locked at one position, and holding that single spot opened processing deeper than anything their faster work had produced. Grand followed the anomaly the way Shapiro had followed hers. The result became Brainspotting, organized around a single memorable claim: where you look affects how you feel (Grand, 2013).

Brainspotting kept EMDR's conviction that the visual system is a doorway to unprocessed material, and changed nearly everything else. Movement became stillness. The tight protocol loosened into an attuned, client-led process in which the therapist finds the relevant eye position, sometimes called a brainspot, and then largely gets out of the way while the client's brain and body process whatever surfaces, often with little or no talking. Grand and colleagues later proposed that a fixed gaze engages midbrain systems involved in orientation, giving sustained access to subcortical activation that moving eyes pass over (Corrigan & Grand, 2013; Corrigan et al., 2015).

Run the Inheritance Test again. Brainspotting was invented at the exact place where EMDR's structure met its limits, in the office of a clinician whose caseload included deeply traumatized people for whom the standard pace was too much or the words never came. So it is at its best precisely there: material without narrative, clients who process somatically, situations where less direction means more depth. And its inheritance predicts its own strain, because a method born from clinical intuition rather than protocol standardization would spend its first decades rich in testimony and comparatively poor in large controlled trials. Chapter 6 weighs exactly that ledger.

Further Down the Brain

The third branch begins with a question rather than an accident. Frank Corrigan, a psychiatrist in Scotland, had spent years co-authoring the papers that tried to explain why Brainspotting worked, and the explanations kept pointing below the limbic system, down into the brainstem, the most ancient part of the brain. Corrigan asked what would happen if a therapy targeted that level directly. His answer, developed with colleagues and published first in theoretical papers and then in clinical form, is Deep Brain Reorienting (Corrigan & Christie-Sands, 2020; Corrigan et al., 2025).

DBR's core idea is that the decisive moment of a traumatic experience happens before the emotion arrives. In the first fractions of a second, the brainstem turns attention toward the threat, the muscles of the neck and face tense, and a physiological shock passes through the system as reality violates expectation. Only after that sequence does fear or horror or grief flood in. DBR proposes that this initial sequence can remain stored at the brainstem level, and that carefully slowing a person's attention onto its traces, the tension, the shock, allows the sequence to complete and release without the client having to relive the story built on top of it. Chapter 7 walks through what this looks like in a session.

The Inheritance Test one final time. DBR was invented by a scientist for the cases that resisted everything else, with particular attention to dissociation and to wounds from earliest attachment relationships. Expect it to shine where stories are unreachable or unbearable, and where shock and disconnection dominate the picture. And expect its inherited strain to be youth itself: a small practitioner base and an evidence file that, however promising, is one well-designed trial deep. That trial, and what it does and does not establish, gets a full chapter.

What Each Method Assumes

Set the three side by side and the family resemblance is obvious. All three accept the Basement Rule from Chapter 1. All three use the body, and especially the visual and orienting systems, as the staircase down. All three were founded on the same disappointment with insight alone. The differences are just as instructive, and the table below is the map you will carry through the rest of the book.

Question	EMDR	Brainspotting	DBR
Born	1987, research culture	2003, clinical practice	Late 2010s, neuroscience
Primary target	The distressing memory	Felt activation in the body	Brainstem shock sequence

Question	EMDR	Brainspotting	DBR
Eyes	Moving, bilateral	Fixed on one position	Natural orienting, slowed
Structure	High, eight phases	Low, client led	Moderate, sequence led
Talking required	Moderate	Minimal	Minimal
Evidence base	Largest, guideline endorsed	Growing, smaller trials	Early, first trial promising

Auguste learned the cost of ignoring this map. After a difficult year he picked a therapy the way most people do, from a persuasive advertisement, and spent four months in a highly structured protocol while the thing that actually troubled him, a wordless dread with no memory attached, never once came into range. Nobody was at fault. A structured, memory-targeted method had been pointed at a problem with no memory address. When he later understood the family tree, his reaction was not anger but relief, and a better-aimed second attempt. His first choice had failed the Inheritance Test, not him.

> **Action Challenge:** *Before the detailed chapters, commit to a gut ranking in writing. Order the three therapies by pure first impression, one to three, and add one sentence about why. Seal it in the back of your notebook. In Chapter 10 you will compare it against your evidence-based ranking, and the gap between the two lists is often the most instructive thing in the whole exercise.*

Reading the Field Around Them

Two honest notes before the tour begins. First, these three are not the only serious trauma treatments. Somatic experiencing works the body without the visual doorway (Levine, 1997). Sensorimotor psychotherapy integrates movement and posture (Ogden et al., 2006). Trauma-focused cognitive approaches remain first-line recommendations in many guidelines. If your eventual practitioner draws on several, that is a feature of mature clinical work, not a betrayal of any brand.

Second, lineage cuts both ways. Because Brainspotting descends from EMDR, and DBR from the effort to explain Brainspotting, many practitioners are trained in more than one branch, and the boundaries in real offices are softer than the boundaries in books. You are not choosing a nation to pledge allegiance to. You are choosing a starting doorway, with a professional who can move between rooms if your needs change. Hold the map firmly and the borders lightly.

> **Action Challenge:** *One piece of observation this week. Notice a moment when your own difficulty announces itself, and ask a single question: does this trouble have a clear memory address, or is it a felt state with no story attached? Write down the answer. No other single observation will do more to narrow your choice among these three doorways.*

Before You Turn the Page

Three accidents of history produced three living methods. A researcher's walk produced structure and the strongest evidence file in the field. A clinician's wobbling session produced stillness, attunement, and access to the wordless. A scientist's unanswered question produced a therapy aimed at the half second before feeling begins. Each inherited the strengths of its birth and the strains of it, and the Inheritance Test lets you read both in advance. Now we slow down and enter each room properly, starting with the eldest. Chapter 3 seats you in the client's chair for EMDR, from the first intake question to the final body scan.

Chapter 3: EMDR From the Client Chair

Your first appointment is nothing like the videos. You arrive braced for eye movements and difficult memories, and instead you spend an hour talking through your history while the therapist takes careful notes and asks what helps you feel steady. No processing happens at all. If you did not know better, you might think you had wandered into ordinary counseling. You have actually entered the first phase of one of the most deliberately structured therapies ever built, and the structure you cannot yet see is the reason the difficult work, when it comes, will be survivable.

This chapter walks you through EMDR from the inside, in the order you would live it. The aim is not to train you in the method. It is to replace the dramatized version in your head with the real shape of the thing, because you cannot judge the fit of a therapy you have only seen in fiction.

Eight Phases, Plainly

EMDR is organized into eight phases, and knowing them turns a mysterious process into a predictable one (Shapiro, 2012, 2018). Phase one is history and treatment planning, the conversation just described, where you and the therapist map what happened, what troubles you now, and which memories will become targets. Phase two is preparation, and it deserves more respect than it gets. Here you build the skills that keep processing inside your window of tolerance: a calm-place exercise, grounding techniques, an agreed stop signal that puts you in control. For people with complex histories, this phase may last weeks, and a therapist who rushes it is showing you a red flag you will learn to read in Chapter 11.

Phases three through six are the processing engine. You bring up a specific target memory along with its worst image, the negative belief attached to it, and where you feel it in your body, and you rate its disturbance on a simple zero-to-ten scale. Then bilateral stimulation begins: your eyes follow the therapist's fingers back and forth, or you hold buzzers that pulse left and right, or tones alternate in your ears. Sets last half a minute or so, and between them the therapist asks only what you noticed. Images shift, feelings move, associations surface. Nobody analyzes anything mid-stream. When the disturbance rating falls to nothing or near it, a chosen positive belief is strengthened in its place, and a body scan checks for residue. Phase seven closes each session so you leave settled, and phase eight reevaluates at the next meeting.

What Bilateral Stimulation Is

The eye movements are the famous part, so let us be precise about them. Bilateral stimulation means any rhythmic, alternating left-right sensory input, visual, tactile, or auditory. It is not hypnosis, you remain fully awake and in control, and it is not exposure in the classic sense of retelling the story over and over. You touch the memory in brief sets while your attention is partly occupied by the stimulation, which is a strange thing to do, and the strangeness turns out to be the point.

The best-supported explanation is disarmingly simple. Working memory, the mental workspace where you hold an image while attending to it, has limited capacity. Tracking a moving target consumes part of that capacity, so the traumatic image you are simultaneously holding becomes less vivid and less emotionally intense, and each time it is put back into storage it is filed in this softened form (van den Hout & Engelhard, 2012). Other researchers have proposed that the alternating stimulation induces a state with similarities to the memory processing of REM sleep (Stickgold, 2002). The mechanisms are still debated; the observed effect, across many trials, is that targeted memories lose disturbance and stay lost, consistent with what memory scientists call reconsolidation, the re-storage of a memory in altered form (Ecker et al., 2012).

A Target From Start to Finish

Theory becomes clearer through a life, so meet Bindi. Two years after a serious road accident, she could not drive past the intersection where it happened, slept badly, and flinched at brake sounds. Talk therapy had helped her mood and changed nothing about the flinch. Her EMDR course began with two sessions of history and preparation, which she privately considered a waste of time until session four proved otherwise.

Processing the accident was harder than she expected. In the third and fourth sessions the memory came back with a vividness that frightened her, and she used her stop signal twice, and once went home feeling stirred up and doubtful. This is the part the success stories skip, and it is ordinary. Her therapist adjusted the pacing, shortened the sets, and spent extra time closing each session. By the sixth session something unceremonious happened: the image of the intersection simply stopped gripping. Her disturbance rating slid to a one and sat there. The belief I am going to die there had quietly become it was terrible and it is over. Ten sessions in total, and the flinch at brake sounds faded over the following month. Not every course of EMDR ends this cleanly, as the next chapter will show, but this is what the method looks like when the problem and the tool are matched: a single-incident trauma with a clear address, processed to completion.

Notice what the structure gave her. She always knew what phase she was in, what the ratings meant, and that she held a stop signal. I call this the Structure Dividend, the named principle of this chapter: in trauma work, predictable structure is not bureaucracy, it is a safety technology that lets a frightened nervous system take risks it could not otherwise afford. Some people find EMDR's structure confining. Many more find it is precisely what makes the descent bearable. Which kind of person you are is a genuine datum for your decision, and no one can supply it but you.

> **Action Challenge:** *A writing task. Draft the opening you would give in a phase-one history session: five to ten sentences covering what happened in broad strokes, what troubles you most now, and what steadies you. You are not obliged to show it to anyone. People who arrive at a first session having thought this through report that the intake feels collaborative instead of interrogative, whichever therapy they ultimately choose.*

How Long It Takes and What It Costs

Honest numbers, held loosely. For a single distressing event in an otherwise stable life, published protocols and clinical experience suggest meaningful change is often possible within roughly six to twelve sessions, sometimes fewer. For complex or repeated trauma, the arc is longer, commonly months rather than weeks, with a substantial preparation phase before processing begins in earnest (Gonzalez-Vazquez et al., 2018). Sessions typically run sixty to ninety minutes. Costs vary widely by region and practitioner, and some public health systems and insurers cover EMDR precisely because of its guideline status, which is worth checking before you assume it is out of reach.

Two practical notes complete the picture. EMDR is delivered by telehealth routinely now, with bilateral stimulation adapted to the screen, and research on remote delivery has generally been reassuring. And the method has spawned variations, including intensives that compress work into consecutive days, and protocol updates such as EMDR 2.0 that deliberately increase the working-memory load (Matthijssen et al., 2021). Treat variations as questions to ask a prospective therapist, not as decisions to make alone.

> **Action Challenge:** *A conversation task. Tell one trusted person what you learned about how EMDR actually proceeds, the eight phases, the preparation, the stop signal. Teaching a thing in plain words is the fastest test of whether you understand it, and saying*

> *your options aloud to another human being is quietly one of the most clarifying acts in this whole process.*

What to Carry Forward

EMDR is a structured, eight-phase therapy that touches specific memories in brief sets while taxing working memory with bilateral stimulation, until the memories are re-stored with their disturbance drained. Its preparation phase is a load-bearing wall, its structure is a safety technology, and its natural home is trauma with a clear address. You have now seen its best case in Bindi, including the rough patch her success story would normally omit. The next chapter holds the method up to honest light: the strength of its evidence, the edges of its reach, and the people it frustrates, because a fair comparison needs the strains as much as the shine.

Chapter 4: EMDR Under Honest Light

Here is a sentence that sounds like an attack and is actually just arithmetic. The best-evidenced trauma therapy in the world leaves a large share of the people who try it without sufficient relief. Both halves are true at once. EMDR's evidence file is the strongest of the three methods in this book, and reviews of trauma treatment as a whole report nonresponse rates that should humble every method on the shelf (Lewis, Roberts, Andrew, et al., 2020; Schottenbauer et al., 2008). If you hold only the first half, you become a salesperson. If you hold only the second, you become a cynic. This chapter asks you to hold both, because both are what you will be standing on when you choose.

The Strength Nobody Disputes

Start with what EMDR has earned. Randomized controlled trials, the demanding kind with comparison groups, have tested it for decades, and systematic reviews consistently find it effective for post-traumatic stress, on par with the best trauma-focused cognitive approaches (Bisson et al., 2013; Watkins et al., 2018). On the strength of that file, it is recommended in the clinical guidelines of the World Health Organization, the American Psychological Association, and the United Kingdom's national health guidance, among others (World Health Organization, 2013; American Psychological Association, 2017; National Institute for Health and Care Excellence, 2018). No other therapy in this book can say anything comparable, and it matters practically as well as scientifically: guideline status is often what persuades an insurer or public health service to pay.

It is worth being precise about what this evidence covers best. The trials that built EMDR's reputation leaned heavily on adults with post-traumatic stress from identifiable events. Within that territory, the method is about as validated as psychotherapy gets. The honest questions begin at the borders of that territory, and borders are exactly what a chooser needs mapped. That is the named principle of this chapter, the Edge Map: the most useful thing you can know about any treatment is not its center, where everyone agrees it works, but its edges, where it starts to strain, because your decision is only hard if you live near an edge.

Where the Protocol Strains

Three edges appear again and again in research and clinical writing. The first is complexity. When trauma was repeated, prolonged, or began in childhood, the tidy picture of one target memory processed to completion gives way to networks of interlocking material, and standard protocols need extension and modification. Clinicians working with severely traumatized clients describe long stabilization phases before processing can safely begin, and structured adaptations exist precisely because the unmodified approach was not enough (Gonzalez-Vazquez et al., 2018; Herman, 1992).

The second edge is dissociation. EMDR's processing phases ask you to hold a target in dual attention, one foot in the memory and one in the room. A nervous system whose signature move is to disconnect can find that task nearly impossible: the buzzers buzz, the fingers move, and the person is no longer present enough for anything to integrate. This is workable, with extended preparation and clinicians trained in dissociation, but it is genuine work against the grain of the method (Lanius et al., 2010).

The third edge is material with no address. The protocol begins by selecting a target memory, which quietly assumes there is one. Trauma encoded before language, or stored as pure body state, offers the protocol nothing to aim at. Skilled practitioners have workarounds, targeting the felt sense or the earliest available fragment, and sometimes they succeed. But you are watching a structured method improvise at its border, and the two younger therapies in this book were both born, in part, at exactly this spot.

The Intensity Question

Then there is the experience itself. EMDR processes by contacting the material, and contact costs. Some people describe sessions as the hardest hours of their year, and a between-session stirring of dreams, emotion, and memory fragments is common enough that good clinicians warn you about it in advance. For a person with a wide window of tolerance this is a fair price paid briefly. For a person with a narrow window it can tip into flooding, the state where activation exceeds what can be integrated, and repeated flooding is not therapy, it is rehearsal of overwhelm.

Two things keep this honest rather than alarming. First, the method contains its own counterweights: the preparation phase, the stop signal, the closing procedures, the therapist's obligation to keep the work inside your window. Flooding in well-conducted EMDR is a pacing failure, not a design feature. Second, intensity is not uniform across people or even across sessions, as Bindi's wobble in the last chapter showed. The question for your framework is not whether EMDR is too intense in general. It is whether your window, as you observed it in Chapter 1's tally, can hold brief, structured contact with your worst material when the structure is working properly.

Two Lives at the Edges

Ephie's history was not one event but a childhood's worth, and her EMDR course showed it. Preparation went well, but each attempt at processing opened not a memory but a cascade, one scene pulling ten others behind it, and twice she left sessions more activated than she arrived. Around session nine, by agreement, she and her therapist paused the processing work entirely. It would be easy to file her under failure, and wrong. What she gained was a precise picture of her own system: complex material, a narrow window, a strong pull toward shutdown under load. She did not yet have relief. She had coordinates, and coordinates are what Part III of this book turns into decisions.

Cashel stood at a different edge with a different outcome. His trauma had an address, but his tendency to disconnect made standard processing slippery, so his therapist shifted to an attachment-informed, heavily paced adaptation: shorter sets, more grounding, months of it. Progress came, and came slowly, and plateaued somewhere real but partial. His sleep recovered and his relationships eased; a residue of numbness stayed. He describes the work as worth it and incomplete, which is a sentence you should get comfortable hearing, because honest trauma treatment produces it often.

> **Action Challenge:** *A writing task that becomes a tool. Open a page with three headings: Complexity, Dissociation, Address. Under each, write two or three sentences locating yourself. One event or many years? Do you flood, disconnect, or both? Does your trouble have a nameable memory, or only a felt state? This page is the first column of the fit scorecard you will complete for all three therapies, and it converts this chapter's edges from information into instrument.*

Adaptations Worth Asking About

The field has not stood still at its edges, and a chooser should know the names of the workarounds. Attachment-focused EMDR extends preparation and weaves relational repair through the protocol for developmental trauma. The progressive approach, developed for complex trauma and dissociation, sequences the work gradually and has controlled research behind it (Gonzalez-Vazquez et al., 2018). Intensive formats compress treatment into consecutive days for people who do better with immersion than weekly drip. And EMDR

2.0 sharpens the working-memory mechanism itself, adding demands that further blunt a memory's vividness during processing, with early comparative research suggesting the added load does what the theory predicts (Matthijssen et al., 2021).

The practical use of this list is not to make you an expert in any adaptation. It is to upgrade your questions. A prospective therapist who hears complex childhood trauma and answers with a plan, extended stabilization, an adapted protocol, a rationale, is showing you the Edge Map in action. One who offers the standard eight phases for every history has not read their own method's borders, and Chapter 11 will teach you to keep interviewing.

> **Action Challenge:** *An observation task for the week. Notice one moment when you were offered a one-size answer to a personal problem, in any domain of life, and how it landed. You are training the exact instinct this book keeps sharpening: the difference between a good tool and a good fit, which no amount of tool quality can erase.*

Where This Leaves You

EMDR enters your comparison with the strongest credentials on the table and three honestly mapped edges: complexity, dissociation, and material without an address, plus an intensity profile that demands respect for your window of tolerance. If your difficulty lives near its center, a discrete trauma, a nameable memory, a system that can stay present under structure, it has earned the right to be your leading candidate. If you recognized yourself in Ephie or Cashel, hold your place. The next two chapters enter the room that was built, almost literally, for the people EMDR's edges frustrate: a quieter room, a fixed gaze, and a therapy that asks the body to lead.

Chapter 5: Where You Look Matters

The room is quieter than you expect a therapy room to be. No fingers sweep across your visual field, no buzzers pulse in your palms. The therapist holds a thin pointer, moves it slowly, and watches your face with unhurried attention. Somewhere left of center your breath catches, a small thing you would never have noticed alone, and the pointer stops. Hold there, she says. You hold there. For a long time nobody speaks, and under the stillness something in your chest begins, very slowly, to move.

That is Brainspotting from the inside, and its texture is the first thing to understand about it. Where EMDR is a procedure you go through, Brainspotting is closer to a state you are held in. Both aim at the basement. They take different staircases, and this chapter walks you down the second one.

A Different Kind of Session

A Brainspotting session usually begins with a simple act of focusing. You bring to mind the issue you want to work on, not necessarily a memory, sometimes only a feeling, a body sensation, a stuckness, and notice how activated you feel and where you sense it physically. Then comes the distinctive step: finding the eye position that connects to that activation. The therapist may track your eyes slowly across your field of vision and stop where something visibly shifts, a blink, a wobble, a change in breathing, which practitioners call the outside window. Or you may be asked where it feels most intense as your gaze moves, called the inside window. Some spots are found from where you spontaneously stare when talking about hard things, called gazespotting. The names matter less than the shared idea: a particular fixed eye position corresponds to the activation you brought, and holding it keeps a channel open (Grand, 2013).

What follows looks, from the outside, like almost nothing. You rest your gaze on the spot, often along the pointer, sometimes with soft bilateral sound in headphones, and you attend to whatever unfolds inside: sensations, images, emotions, memories, or long stretches of wordless shifting. The therapist speaks little. There is no protocol demanding you rate anything, retrieve anything, or report between sets. Sessions commonly run fifty to ninety minutes, and people often describe time distorting, the way it does in deep concentration.

Why a Fixed Gaze

The proposed mechanism runs through the brain's orienting system. Where your eyes point is controlled by ancient midbrain circuitry, including the superior colliculus, that also participates in threat detection and bodily state. Corrigan and Grand argued that a sustained, relevant eye position gives prolonged access to subcortical activation, letting sensorimotor memory be contacted and processed at a level beneath narrative, and that stillness reaches what movement passes over (Corrigan & Grand, 2013; Corrigan et al., 2015). The theory remains a theory, further along than folklore and well short of proven, and Chapter 6 will treat it with the same scales we used on EMDR.

The second half of the method is not optical at all. Grand calls it the dual attunement frame: the therapist attunes simultaneously to the brainspot and to you, tracking your face, breath, and micro-signals with full attention. Practitioners consider this attunement half the treatment, and it explains something the diagrams cannot, which is why clients so often describe feeling accompanied at depths where they had always been alone. A method with almost no talking turns out to be intensely relational.

The Quiet Doorway

Now the named principle of this chapter, and the reason this room exists. I call it the Quiet Doorway: some material can only be reached by a method that does not require you to speak it, because the material was never stored in words to begin with. Chapter 1 established that trauma can be encoded as fragments and body states. Chapter 4 showed a structured, verbal, memory-targeted protocol straining at exactly that edge. Brainspotting is what a therapy looks like when it is designed on the other side of that edge, asking nothing of language and everything of attention.

Alora's history makes the principle concrete. Hospitalized repeatedly before her third birthday, she grew up with a body that treated clinics, and eventually most enclosed rooms, as emergencies, while her explicit memory of those years held nothing at all. Talk therapy had given her understanding and no traction; there was no story to tell, only a state that arrived. In Brainspotting she never had to produce one. Session after session she held a spot low and to the right while her body worked through waves of heat, pressure, and, once, twenty minutes of shaking that resolved into an unfamiliar calm. Progress was real and jagged. The clinic response softened over four months; a stubborn residue around one specific smell did not budge, and she and her practitioner eventually folded in other somatic work for it. Partial, meaningful, honest: remember her arc when the testimonials you meet online promise miracles.

> **Action Challenge:** *An observation task, with a boundary attached. This week, simply notice where your eyes go when you are stressed, that you stare at corners, floors, or middle distance, and that some resting places feel different from others. Notice only. Do not attempt to hold positions and process on yourself; this is a relational therapy for good reasons, and self-experimentation with traumatic activation is how people get flooded alone. Curiosity now, practitioners later.*

What the Body Leads

Because the client's process leads, Brainspotting bends to an unusual range of uses. Practitioners work with trauma, anxiety, grief, chronic pain presentations, and performance blocks in athletes and performers, the last being an area Grand himself developed extensively (Grand, 2013). The method's flexibility is genuine and it cuts both ways, which deserves saying plainly. The same openness that lets a wordless history unfold can leave a person who thrives on structure feeling unmoored, unsure what is happening or whether anything is. In the next chapter you will meet Tovey, for whom the quiet felt not like a doorway but like a waiting room, and his experience is as much data as Alora's.

Expectations, honestly set: Brainspotting sessions are often described as gentler than EMDR at the moment of contact, with activation rising and falling in tolerable waves, and it still stirs material between sessions, still requires a window of tolerance, and still deserves the same preparation conversation any deep work deserves. Gentler is not gentle. It is a different distribution of the same necessary cost.

> **Action Challenge:** *A writing task for your scorecard. Answer in a paragraph: when you have made real progress on anything difficult, did it come through structure, plans, steps, and measurable targets, or through space, immersion, and following what emerged? Neither answer is better. One of them is yours, and the difference between this chapter's room and the last one's turns largely on it.*

The Part Worth Keeping

Brainspotting holds the eyes still where EMDR moves them, follows the body where EMDR follows the protocol, and treats deep attunement as half the medicine. Its doorway is quiet on purpose, built for material that language cannot carry, and its openness will feel like freedom to some readers and like fog to others. You now know what the room is like. The next chapter asks the harder question of what the evidence actually shows, who tends to thrive here, who walks away, and what those certification levels behind a practitioner's name really mean.

Chapter 6: Brainspotting Weighed and Measured

Put the method on trial. The charge, made by skeptics, is that Brainspotting is testimony all the way down, a compelling experience with thin proof. The defense answers with two decades of clinical results and a growing stack of studies. Your job in this chapter is to be neither prosecutor nor defense but the judge, because you are the one who has to act on the verdict, and acting on someone else's verdict is how mismatches happen.

Begin with the principle that organizes everything here. I call it the Evidence Ladder: treatments are not simply proven or unproven, they stand on rungs, from anecdote at the bottom, through case series and small comparative studies, up to large randomized trials and the systematic reviews that pool them. A method's rung tells you how much confidence its claims have earned so far. It does not tell you whether the method will help you, and confusing those two questions ruins more treatment decisions than any other single error.

What the Studies Show

Brainspotting's file is real and modest, and both words matter. The most direct comparison came from a study of seventy-six adults seeking help after traumatic events, treated with three sessions of either EMDR or Brainspotting under standard protocols. Both groups improved significantly. Reported effect sizes on post-traumatic symptoms ran larger for EMDR, roughly 1.19 to 1.76 across measures, against roughly 0.74 to 1.04 for Brainspotting, with the authors concluding that Brainspotting appears to be an effective alternative (Hildebrand et al., 2017). For scale, effect sizes near 0.8 are conventionally called large, so the honest summary is two effective treatments, with the older one showing somewhat stronger numbers in this sample.

A second line of evidence compared single forty-minute sessions of EMDR, Brainspotting, and body scan meditation for distressing memories in a nonclinical sample of forty health professionals. Both EMDR and Brainspotting reduced disturbance immediately and at follow-up weeks later, with some differences in how each affected the way memories were recounted (D'Antoni et al., 2022). Smaller studies and case series report benefits for anxiety, post-traumatic symptoms, and other conditions, and reviewers consistently add the same caveat: samples are small, designs vary, and replication by independent teams is thin. One thoughtful critic put it plainly, that the research base remains weak for a method of its age, with low-powered studies open to therapist influence.

Place all this on the ladder. Brainspotting stands on the middle rungs: controlled comparative evidence exists and points the right way, while the large multi-site trials and systematic reviews that carried EMDR into international guidelines have not yet been done. That is a fair, unglamorous position for a therapy of its generation, better evidenced than most of what circulates under the trauma healing banner, and short of the standard its older sibling has set.

The Fair Criticism and the Fair Reply

The criticism deserves its full weight, so give it. Small samples overstate effects. Studies run by practitioners invested in a method are vulnerable to bias, however honest the practitioners. A theory about midbrain access, elegant as the papers are, is not itself evidence of outcomes (Corrigan et al., 2015). And a treatment popular for twenty years could, in principle, have organized the definitive trial by now. Anyone who waves this away is selling something.

The fair reply is about how evidence actually gets made. Large trials follow money and institutions, and Brainspotting grew up in private practice, outside the university and pharmaceutical structures that fund definitive studies. Absence of large trials under those conditions is weak evidence of absence. Meanwhile the mechanism question is being worked from the neuroscience side by serious researchers, and the comparative studies that do exist found genuine effects, not noise. The judge's summary: promising, plausible, under-tested, improving. Now the question that actually decides things, which is not how strong the evidence is in general, but who the method serves.

Who Tends to Thrive and Who Walks Away

Hemi arrived at Brainspotting after structured therapy kept sliding off him. His difficulty had no single address, he went quiet under pressure rather than loud, and being asked to narrate had always felt like translating from a language he did not speak. The quiet room fit him almost immediately. Across five months he processed in long wordless stretches, and the change showed up first in his body, sleep, jaw, the disappearance of a permanent low dread, before he had any story about why. He still keeps a monthly session. He calls it maintenance; his practitioner calls it consolidation; either way, it is the picture of a method matched to a nervous system.

Tovey walked away, and his account deserves equal standing. An engineer by temperament as much as trade, he wanted to know what was happening, how progress would be measured, and what came next, and the open process gave him nothing to hold. Sessions felt like sitting in a waiting room for a train nobody would confirm. After eight weeks he stopped, not in crisis, simply unconvinced, and later did well in a far more structured therapy. Nothing malfunctioned. A man who runs on structure met the one room in this book with the least of it, and the Inheritance Test from Chapter 2 could have predicted the result before a single session was paid for.

> **Action Challenge:** *A writing task. Complete the Brainspotting column of your scorecard with three short answers. Does my difficulty have an address, or is it felt state, Chapter 2's question, now with a room attached. Did my honest answer in Chapter 5 favor structure or space. And where did my sympathies land between Hemi and Tovey, because that reaction is itself data.*

Certification, Decoded

Because you will eventually read practitioner profiles, learn the labels now. Brainspotting training proceeds in phases. Phase one teaches the fundamentals, outside and inside window, basic setup. Phase two adds advanced techniques and deepens the attunement work. Later phases and specialty trainings extend the method further, and a separate certification credential requires accumulated training, consultation hours, and practice. The practical translation: phases completed tell you exposure to the method, certification tells you supervised depth in it. For trauma work, and especially for complex histories, you want depth, and Chapter 11 will script the exact questions that establish it politely.

One more label matters here. Because Brainspotting is unregulated as a term, anyone from a psychologist to a coach can complete trainings and advertise it. The trainings are open by design, which widens access and widens variance. Your protection is boring and effective: verify the underlying license first, the mental health qualification that makes someone accountable to a professional board, and treat Brainspotting credentials as a specialty layered on top, never as a substitute.

> **Action Challenge:** *A conversation task. Find one person in your circle who has tried any somatic or brain-based therapy and ask two questions only: what did a session actually feel like, and what do you wish you had known first. You are not gathering verdicts, you are calibrating expectations, and secondhand texture from someone you trust beats a hundred anonymous reviews.*

One Thing to Hold

If this chapter leaves you with a single sentence, take this one: Brainspotting is a middle-rung therapy with real comparative evidence behind it, a plausible but unproven mechanism, and a fit profile so distinct that the same room produced Hemi's quiet recovery and Tovey's polite exit. Judge it by rung and by fit together, never by either alone. Now we descend the last staircase. The youngest therapy in this book was built by asking what happens in the half second before fear itself, and to understand it you will need to slow a single moment down until it almost stops.

Chapter 7: The Therapy Beneath the Story

Slow one moment down until it almost stops. A person steps off a curb and a horn blares. Before fear, before thought, before any possibility of words, a sequence fires. The head and eyes snap toward the sound. The muscles of the neck and shoulders seize to move the head and brace it. And through the middle of the body runs a jolt, the physiological thud of a world that has just violated its own predictions. All of that happens in well under a second. The fear arrives afterward, and the story after that, and the retelling at dinner after that. Deep Brain Reorienting begins with a radical act of attention: it ignores the dinner version, largely ignores even the fear, and goes looking for the snap, the seize, and the thud.

The Half Second Before Fear

The developers of DBR call this firing order the orienting sequence, and mapping it in plain language is the fastest way to understand the therapy. First comes orienting: ancient midbrain circuitry turns attention toward anything sudden or significant, and it does so before the thinking brain knows anything has happened. Second comes orienting tension: the physical component, felt mostly in the neck, shoulders, face, and around the eyes, as the body organizes to face the thing. Third comes shock: a rapid, whole-system jolt when what is happening cannot be reconciled with what was expected, the gasp made flesh. Only fourth comes affect, the tidal wave of fear, horror, helplessness, or grief that most therapies treat as the beginning of the traumatic response (Corrigan & Christie-Sands, 2020).

DBR's founding claim is that in overwhelming events, this sequence can fail to complete and discharge, leaving its residue held at the level of the brainstem, beneath emotion, beneath memory as we usually mean it, beneath every floor that talking reaches. If that is where the residue lives, the argument runs, that is where therapy should go. I call this chapter's named principle the Shock Before the Story: the deepest layer of a traumatic imprint is often not the memory or even the emotion but the interrupted physical sequence that preceded both, and a therapy aimed at that layer needs neither the story nor the flood to do its work.

Notice how directly this claim descends from the previous chapters. Chapter 1 put trauma in the basement. EMDR works the basement through memory, Brainspotting through felt activation. DBR says there is a subbasement, and its founder should know, since he spent years co-authoring the theoretical papers on why Brainspotting reaches as deep as it does before concluding that something lay deeper still (Corrigan & Grand, 2013; Corrigan et al., 2025).

Inside a DBR Session

The experience is slower and stranger than either room you have visited so far. You and the therapist choose not a memory to process but an activating cue, sometimes a brief thought of a difficult person or moment, sometimes an image, sometimes barely more than a word. The cue is touched lightly, and then the therapy's real question is asked: what happens in your neck, your shoulders, your face, around your eyes. Not what do you feel emotionally. What tenses. You are being guided to notice the orienting tension, the second step of the sequence, and to stay with it at a level of patience that most people have never applied to their own body.

What follows is tracked in sensations. The tension may sharpen, shift, or reveal a deeper layer; at some point many people contact something harder to describe, a dropping, a jolt, a wave through the chest or stomach, which the model identifies as the held shock beginning to move. The therapist's job is pacing: keeping the process slow enough that the sequence can complete this time, in safety, in order, without tipping into the emotional flood that sits above it. Sessions are quiet, largely wordless in their middle stretches, and clients often report that very little seemed to happen until they noticed, days later, that something chronic had unclenched. Retelling is not required at any point. The story may surface, and may be spoken about afterward, but the method does not run on it.

Zowie's course shows the shape. Her difficulty traced to a sudden abandonment in early adolescence, and years of capable talk therapy had rendered the story inert on the upper floors while a bodily bracing, throat, jaw, a permanent slight flinch from closeness, never left. In DBR she barely told the story at all. Session after session she tracked the tension around her eyes and the strange heaviness that followed it, and across four months the bracing loosened in increments she could measure in unguarded moments with people she loved. It did not finish the work; grief surfaced as the bracing left, and she took the grief to a therapist who works with exactly that. She describes DBR as the thing that unlocked the door rather than the thing that furnished the room, which is about as precise a review as a new therapy could ask for.

Built With Dissociation in Mind

One design feature deserves its own section, because for some readers it is the whole argument. The clinical writing behind DBR gives sustained attention to dissociation and to attachment wounding, the injuries formed in the earliest relationships, and the method's mechanics show it (Corrigan et al., 2025). By working beneath the emotional level, at tension and shock rather than at the flood itself, DBR is built to stay under the intensity that typically triggers disconnection. The pacing is titrated by design. There is no dual-attention task to fail, no narrative to produce, no requirement to hold a memory steady while the system is begging to leave.

None of this makes it effortless or universally gentle; contacting held shock is strange, sometimes intense, and requires the same relational safety as everything else in this book. But if Chapter 4's dissociation edge described you, if you are the person who departs rather than floods, you should recognize what you are looking at: a therapy whose founding papers treat your response not as an obstacle to the method but as a central design constraint. That is rare, and in your framework it will count.

> **Action Challenge:** *An observation task, with the same boundary as Chapter 5's. Once or twice this week, in an ordinary moment of stress, a sharp email, a near miss in traffic, notice afterward what your neck, shoulders, and face did, and in what order things seemed to happen. You are learning to perceive the orienting tension this chapter described, nothing more. Do not go hunting for shock or pair this noticing with traumatic material on your own; that is precisely the work that belongs in a paced, professional setting.*

What It Is Not

Three boundaries keep the picture accurate. DBR is not a relaxation technique; the stillness is instrumental, aimed at completion of a specific sequence, and sessions can contact very deep material. It is not a shortcut that replaces grieving, meaning-making, or the rebuilding of a life, as Zowie's handoff showed; it addresses a particular layer, and layers above it may still need their own work. And it is not yet a widely available commodity: the practitioner base is small, trainings are recent, and finding someone may take real effort, a practical constraint the next chapter weighs alongside the evidence. What it is, distinctly, is the only therapy in this book aimed at the half second before feeling begins.

The Takeaway Plainly

DBR targets the brainstem's interrupted first response, orienting, tension, shock, and helps it complete without requiring the story or the flood. It descends directly from the effort to explain Brainspotting, was designed with dissociation and earliest wounds in view, and trades breadth of availability for depth of target. You have now stood in all three rooms. Before the head-to-head comparison, one more piece of due diligence remains, the same one you performed twice already: what the evidence for this young method actually shows, what interim means, and what an honest early adopter's ledger looks like.

Chapter 8: DBR and the Early Evidence

A report from the field, dated 2023. A research team in Canada, led by trauma neuroscientists and including DBR's developer, published the first randomized controlled trial of the method in the European Journal of Psychotraumatology. Fifty-four adults with post-traumatic stress disorder were randomly assigned to eight sessions of DBR delivered by videoconference or to a waitlist. The treated group showed significant decreases in symptoms at the end of treatment and again at three-month follow-up, and attrition was strikingly low, with a single participant not completing treatment (Kearney et al., 2023). For a therapy barely out of its founding papers, it is about as strong an opening statement as the format allows.

Your job in this chapter is the same judging work you did for Brainspotting, with one added skill: reading early evidence without either inflating it or dismissing it. Both errors are common, both are expensive, and the tool for avoiding them is this chapter's named principle. I call it the Early Adopter Ledger: when a treatment is young, write its promise on one page and its unknowns on the facing page, and make no decision until both pages are full. Enthusiasts read only the left page. Cynics read only the right. Choosers read the spread.

The Left Page

Enter the promise honestly, because there is real promise to enter. The trial was randomized and controlled, the design that earns middle-to-upper rungs on the Evidence Ladder, and its effects held at follow-up rather than evaporating. The near-absence of dropout matters more than it may look: trauma treatments as a class lose a meaningful share of participants, and a method people can stay in is solving one of the field's quietest problems (Lewis, Roberts,

Andrew, et al., 2020). Delivery by videoconference matters practically too, since it means the trial's version of DBR is the version a reader far from any major city could actually receive.

Add the deeper entries. DBR is unusual among young therapies in being theory-first: it arrived with a specified neural target and published scientific rationale before its outcome trial, rather than assembling explanations after the fact (Corrigan & Christie-Sands, 2020). The research group has framed the interim results as showing effectiveness in the range of established treatments while calling for larger studies, an unusually careful public posture. And the method's design attention to dissociation gives it a candidate role for exactly the population that mainstream protocols serve least well, which is where new treatments earn their keep.

The Right Page

Now the unknowns, entered with equal care. One trial is one trial. Its sample was modest, its comparison was a waitlist rather than an active established therapy, and waitlist comparisons flatter every treatment, since doing something structured reliably beats doing nothing. No independent replication by teams unconnected to the method's developers has yet been published. Durability beyond three months, performance against EMDR head-to-head, results across different trauma types and severities, and the neuroimaging confirmation of the proposed mechanism all remain open questions, and the trial authors said so themselves (Kearney et al., 2023).

Add the practical unknowns, which for you may weigh more. The practitioner base is small and unevenly spread, trainings are recent, and there is no long-established certification ecosystem of the kind EMDR has built over decades. Public guidelines do not yet mention DBR, which means insurers and health systems mostly will not fund it. And a young method's variance problem is real: with fewer practitioners and less accumulated supervision culture, the gap between the best and worst delivery of DBR is likely wider than for its elders. None of this is disqualifying. All of it belongs on the page.

Reading the Spread

Hold both pages and the honest position writes itself. DBR is a promising, theoretically serious, well-behaved young therapy with one strong trial, no independent replication, and thin availability. If your situation matches its design center, dominant shock and bracing, dissociation, wordless or earliest material, especially if the alternatives have already disappointed you, it is a rational candidate now, chosen with open eyes. If your situation sits comfortably in the center of an established method's map, choosing DBR first means paying an early adopter's premium, in search costs and uncertainty, for depth you may not need. That is not a warning against it. It is the price sheet.

Orson read the spread and paid the premium knowingly. Established treatment had helped his mood and left a core of frozen shock untouched, so when he found a DBR-trained clinician two towns over, he committed to a course and kept notes like the engineer of his own trial. His ledger after five months was genuinely mixed. The chronic bracing through his chest and neck, his oldest companion, released to a degree nothing else had touched, and he called that alone worth the search. His sleep improved partially. A cluster of avoidance habits did not move at all, and he eventually took those to a structured behavioral approach, where they yielded. Asked whether he would choose DBR again, he said yes, and then added the sentence this whole chapter exists to teach: but I would still make the same choice the same way, both pages first.

> **Action Challenge:** *A writing task. Draw the ledger for yourself. Left page: what specifically about DBR's design speaks to your situation, in your own words, no borrowed hype. Right page: which unknowns would actually affect you, availability where you*

> *live, funding, the thinness of the evidence. If your left page is generic and your right page is long, you have your answer for now. If your left page is precise and personal, carry it into Part III with full standing.*

Watching a Method Grow

Because DBR will change faster than anything else in this book, learn to track it rather than freeze it. Further studies from the original group and new sites will appear; the questions to bring to each are the ones you now own. Was there a comparison group, and was it active or waitlist. Who ran the study, developers or independents. How large, how long, how durable. Did dropout stay low outside the founding team's care. A single afternoon with those questions and a search engine, repeated yearly, will keep your picture current long after this book's snapshot ages. Treat that as standing homework for whichever therapy you choose, since all three files are still being written.

> **Action Challenge:** *A conversation task you will reuse in Chapter 11. Draft the three questions you would ask any DBR practitioner before booking: where they trained in the method and how recently, what their consultation or supervision arrangement looks like, and how they decide DBR is the right tool for a given person rather than the tool they happen to hold. Practitioners who welcome those questions are the ones worth finding.*

What Remains Open

The youngest therapy in this book enters your comparison with one strong trial, a serious theory, remarkable retention, and every large question still open, from replication to availability. You have now done honest due diligence on all three methods, and something useful has happened along the way: you have become the kind of reader who checks pages instead of headlines. What remains is the work this book was named for. In the next chapter, one person carries one difficulty into all three rooms in turn, and the nine lines that truly divide these therapies finally get drawn side by side.

Chapter 9: One Memory, Three Rooms

Run the experiment the field itself has never properly run. Take one person, with one difficulty, and walk them through all three rooms, not as a patient shopping in sequence over disappointing years, but as a thought experiment conducted in a single chapter, holding everything constant except the method. The person is Phaedon, forty-one, a site supervisor. Eleven years ago a scaffold section collapsed beside him, close enough that the impact threw him off his feet; he walked away unmarked and has never since stood comfortably under anything overhead. Crane sounds lock his breath. He sleeps poorly before inspections. He has told the story so many times it bores him, and the telling has never changed the breath.

Phaedon is fictional, assembled from patterns this book has already shown you, and he is about to earn his keep. Watch what each room does with the same man.

The First Room

In the EMDR room, Phaedon's difficulty is a gift to the method: a single incident with a clear address. History-taking maps it in one session; preparation builds his calm place and stop signal in two more, and he is mildly impatient with both until processing begins and he understands. Holding the worst image, the section mid-fall, with the belief I am about to be crushed, he tracks the therapist's fingers in half-minute sets. The memory surges, shifts, throws out associations he had never connected, a childhood fall, his father's yard, and across four processing sessions the disturbance rating walks down from eight to two to a stubborn one that finally releases when a missed fragment, the sound, is targeted directly. The positive belief installed is unremarkable and true: it missed me, and I am careful now. His body scan clears. The crane sounds lose their grip over the following weeks, mostly, and his pre-inspection sleep recovers.

What the room asked of him: sustained contact with the worst of it, trust in a procedure, tolerance for two hard weeks mid-course. What it gave him: measurable, targeted resolution on a schedule, roughly ten sessions. The structure that some find confining fit his difficulty like a jig fits a beam.

The Second Room

In the Brainspotting room, nobody asks Phaedon to hold the worst image. He brings up the scaffold lightly, notices the activation as a band across his chest, and the practitioner tracks his eyes slowly until, high and to the left, his breathing changes. He holds there. What unfolds over the sessions is less linear than the first room and stranger to describe: long silent stretches, waves of heat, a session dominated by trembling through his legs that he later connects to the moment his body wanted to run and had nowhere to go. The story surfaces occasionally and is allowed to pass. Relief arrives less like a rating walking down and more like weather clearing, noticed in retrospect. After four months he stands under the scaffolds fine; the sound sensitivity is perhaps half gone and fades further over the year.

What this room asked of him: tolerance for not knowing where the process was going, comfort with the body leading, patience with progress that resists measurement. What it gave him: depth without direct assault on the memory, and the discharge of a physical urge the first room had touched only in passing. A man who needed structure might have walked out at week three. Phaedon, as it happens, could work either way, which is exactly why he makes a fair test subject.

The Third Room

In the DBR room, the scaffold barely features as a story at all. The cue is a single image held lightly, and the entire opening question is about his neck. Phaedon discovers, to his surprise, that thinking of the site produces an instant seizing across his right shoulder and jaw, the body's memory of wrenching away, and that beneath it, reached slowly across several sessions, sits something he can only call a thud, the shock of the world breaking its promise a half second before any fear he remembers. The work is the slowest of the three and the quietest: tracking tension, letting it sharpen and release, letting the thud move through in increments. He cries once, without images, and cannot say why, and feels lighter for days.

What this room asked of him: extraordinary patience, tolerance for working beneath the level of story entirely, and the search costs of finding the practitioner at all. What it gave him: release of a layer the other rooms addressed indirectly, the bracing itself, with the least contact with distressing content of the three. Had Phaedon been someone who dissociates under any contact with the memory, this room's advantage would have widened from notable to decisive.

The Nine Lines That Divide Them

Now formalize what the three visits showed. I call this chapter's named principle the Nine Dividing Lines: three legitimate therapies for the same wound differ along nine practical dimensions, and your decision lives in those nine lines, not in any global ranking. The table below is the master comparison, and everything in it traces back to chapters you have already read.

Dividing line	EMDR	Brainspotting	DBR
Primary target	Specific memory network	Felt activation in body	Brainstem shock sequence
Structure of sessions	High, protocol driven	Low, client led	Moderate, sequence paced

Dividing line	EMDR	Brainspotting	DBR
Verbal demand	Moderate	Minimal	Minimal
Contact intensity	Highest, direct	Moderate, wave-like	Lowest, beneath affect
Fit with dissociation	Strained, needs adaptation	Good	Designed for it
Preverbal or wordless material	Edge of the map	Strong	Strong
Evidence maturity	Guideline endorsed	Middle rungs	One strong trial
Practitioner availability	Widest	Moderate	Thin
Typical course, single incident	Roughly six to twelve sessions	Weeks to months, variable	Weeks to months, early data

Where They Agree

Do not let the lines hide the common ground, because the common ground is most of the picture. All three rooms healed Phaedon meaningfully. All three worked bottom-up, respected his window of tolerance, and depended, more than any technique, on a skilled and attuned practitioner, a factor Chapter 11 will argue outweighs several lines of this table combined. Comparative research keeps finding that legitimate trauma therapies share effectiveness more than marketing admits (Watkins et al., 2018; D'Antoni et al., 2022). The choice you are making is real and consequential and it is a choice among goods, which should lower the temperature of the deciding considerably.

> **Action Challenge:** *The writing task this chapter was built for. Copy the nine dividing lines onto a page and circle the three that matter most for you, not in general, for you, given everything your notebook now holds: your window tally, your address-or-state answer, your structure-or-space paragraph, your edge locations,*

> *your ledger. Most readers find their circles cluster fast, and clustered circles are a decision most of the way made.*

Standing Between the Rooms

One man, one wound, three legitimate doorways, nine lines of real difference and a wide floor of common ground. If a single winner existed, this chapter is where it would have been crowned, and instead you watched the crown pass from room to room depending on which line you weighted. That is the deepest finding in this entire field, and the next chapter turns it into machinery: five factors, a scoring grid, four special pathways, and three worked decisions, so that the circles on your page become a name on your shortlist.

Chapter 10: The Matching Framework

Look at the person in the mirror for a moment, because they are the subject of this chapter. Not trauma survivors in general, not the average participant in any trial, but the one reader whose notebook now holds a window tally, an address-or-state answer, a structure-or-space paragraph, three edge locations, an early adopter's ledger, and nine dividing lines with three circles on them. Every previous chapter collected evidence about the therapies. This one weighs the evidence about you, and the weighing has a principle behind it that I have been saving for exactly this point.

I call it the Nervous System Vote: in choosing a trauma therapy, your body's demonstrated patterns get a vote equal to the research evidence, because a method your system cannot work inside will fail regardless of its trial results. The trials tell you what works for populations. Your tally, your shutdowns, your floods, your wordless states tell you what your particular system can use. Neither voter should be silenced, and every bad match in this book so far, Auguste's, Ephie's, Tovey's, happened because one of them was.

Five Factors That Decide

Everything you have gathered reduces to five factors. First, trauma type: single incident, complex and repeated, or preverbal and wordless, established by your Chapter 4 page. Second, dominant response pattern: flooding, shutdown and dissociation, or manageable activation, established by your window tally. Third, material address: nameable memory or felt state, your Chapter 2 observation. Fourth, processing style: structure or space, your Chapter 5 paragraph. Fifth, practical access: what is actually available, reachable, and affordable where you live, which the last chapters of this book address in full.

Notice what is not on the list. Which therapy your friend swears by is absent, because their nervous system is not casting your vote. Which method sounds most impressive is absent. And which is newest or oldest is absent, because age enters only through the evidence and availability factors, where it belongs.

Scoring the Grid

Now build the instrument. Draw a grid with the three therapies across the top and the five factors down the side, and score each cell from zero to two: two if the therapy is a strong match for your situation on that factor, one if workable, zero if strained. The chapters have already told you how to score. A complex, dissociative presentation scores DBR and Brainspotting high on factors one and two and standard EMDR lower; a single incident with a clear address flips the first row; a structure-lover raises EMDR on factor four; thin local availability drops DBR on factor five, and so on. The table below shows the pattern logic in compressed form.

Factor favors	EMDR	Brainspotting	DBR
Single incident, clear memory	Strong	Workable	Workable
Complex or preverbal history	Adapted only	Strong	Strong
Flooding pattern	Careful pacing	Strong	Strong
Shutdown and dissociation	Adapted only	Strong	Designed for it
Felt state, no address	Strained	Strong	Strong
Structure preference	Strong	Strained	Workable
Space preference	Workable	Strong	Strong

Factor favors	EMDR	Brainspotting	DBR
Funding and guidelines matter	Strong	Workable	Strained
Wide practitioner choice	Strong	Workable	Strained

Total the columns and you have a ranked shortlist, and one instruction matters more than the arithmetic: rank all three, never just crown one. Availability will test your first choice, and a person holding a ranked list negotiates reality; a person holding a single answer gets stopped by it.

Four Special Pathways

Four situations recur so often they deserve named routes through the grid. The first is the reader for whom EMDR already stalled. Return to how it stalled. If processing kept cascading beyond control, the complexity edge, an adapted EMDR with a complex-trauma specialist and the two body-led rooms both deserve scoring. If you kept leaving the room inside yourself, the dissociation edge, weight DBR and Brainspotting sharply upward. If there was simply nothing to aim at, the address edge, the quiet doorways were built for you. Fit Before Fault, applied literally: the stall pattern is diagnostic gold, not a verdict.

The second pathway is the shutdown-dominant reader, who should read row four of the table as this book's most confident single recommendation. The third is the no-narrative reader, whose material predates words or never formed them; both younger rooms score high, and the choice between them usually falls to factor five and the intensity line from Chapter 9. The fourth is the first-timer with a discrete recent trauma and a steady baseline, for whom standard EMDR's center, structure, evidence, availability, and funding, is a genuinely excellent first door, and this book's earlier warnings about its edges should not scare you off its center.

When Logistics Overrule

Say it plainly, because politeness ruins decisions: a perfect-fit therapy with no reachable practitioner is not an option, it is a wish. If your grid crowns DBR and the nearest trained clinician is a continent away with a full practice, your working first choice is the second name on the list, with the first kept on watch as trainings spread. Telehealth widens the map considerably, all three methods are delivered remotely, and DBR's own trial ran by videoconference, so exhaust the online search before conceding (Kearney et al., 2023). But concede when reality insists. The ranked list exists for exactly this moment, and choosing the reachable good over the unreachable perfect is not settling, it is treatment beginning this year instead of someday.

Money belongs in the same honest light. Guideline status means EMDR is the most likely of the three to be covered by insurers and public systems, which for some readers converts a preference gap into a non-decision. Paying privately for a better-matched method can be worth it; going without treatment while saving for the ideal one rarely is.

Three Worked Decisions

Delyth's grid was almost boring, and boring grids are a blessing. One event two years ago, a clear address, manageable activation, a stated love of structure, and an insurer that covers guideline treatments: EMDR won four factors outright, and she booked it within the month. Her course ran close to Bindi's from Chapter 3, hard middle weeks included, and she finished in eleven sessions. The framework's job is sometimes to confirm the obvious quickly and get out of the way.

Rune's grid crowned DBR clearly, shutdown-dominant, wordless material, and the search then found no trained practitioner within reach and a telehealth waitlist quoted in seasons. He activated his second rank, Brainspotting, with a certified practitioner experienced in dissociation, and put his name on the DBR list anyway. Eight months on, the Brainspotting work has moved real ground, slower than he hoped, and he has kept the watchlist habit from Chapter 8. An imperfect route, chosen with open eyes, already producing change: that is what the framework promises, not perfection.

Meeka's decision turned on a single row. Her history was complex, her pattern flooding rather than shutdown, her address answer emphatically felt state, and her one previous structured therapy had felt like being processed by machinery. Brainspotting's combination of body-led pacing and deep attunement won her grid by a margin, and the first practitioner she consulted failed her interview questions, a story Chapter 11 finishes. The second did not. A year later her progress is substantial and unfinished, and she would circle the same name again.

> **Action Challenge:** *The writing task everything has built toward. Complete your grid now, all fifteen cells, total the columns, and write the ranked list on one page with your one-sentence stall statement from the Introduction at the top. Then the behavior task: within one week, show that page to a qualified professional, your current therapist, your physician, a clinician offering consultations, and ask one question: given my history as you know it, what would you add to this page. You are not surrendering the decision. You are adding the one voter this book cannot supply, someone qualified who knows you.*

Your Ranked Answer

Five factors, one grid, four pathways, three worked lives, and the Nervous System Vote counted in full. Whatever names your page now ranks, notice what you have become since the Introduction: a person choosing among understood options with evidence in both hands, which is the entire transformation this book promised. Two tasks remain, and they are practical ones. The finest method on your list still has to be delivered by a particular human being, and finding, questioning, and choosing that human being is a skill of its own. That skill is next.

Chapter 11: Finding Someone Good

Listen in on two phone calls, because Carwen made both of them in one afternoon and the difference decided her year. The first practitioner answered her question about training with a list of impressive-sounding intensives, dismissed her question about pacing with the assurance that everyone is ready sooner than they think, and offered a package price before asking a single question about her history. The second practitioner asked about her history first, answered the training question with specifics, dates, supervision arrangements, described exactly how the early sessions would establish safety before any processing, and named, unprompted, the circumstances under which she would refer Carwen elsewhere. Same method on both business cards. Barely the same profession on the phone.

This chapter exists because of that gap. Everything you have decided so far assumed the method would be delivered well, and delivery is a variable, not a constant. I call this chapter's named principle the Practitioner Premium: who delivers your therapy affects your outcome as much as which therapy you chose, so the search deserves the same rigor as the choice. Research on psychotherapy has long observed that therapist factors and the quality of the working relationship carry substantial weight in outcomes across methods (Wampold, 2015; Flückiger et al., 2018). Your framework got you to a name on a page. This chapter gets you to a person in a room.

What the Letters Mean

Credentials come in two layers, and the layers do different jobs. The foundation layer is the license: the psychologist, counselor, clinical social worker, psychotherapist, or physician registration that makes someone accountable to a professional board with the power to discipline them. This layer is non-negotiable, and it is the first thing to verify, independently, through the board's own register, before any specialty credential impresses you. The specialty layer sits on top: EMDR basic training versus the deeper certification and consultant designations of its professional associations; Brainspotting's phase trainings versus its accumulated certification, as Chapter 6 decoded; DBR's recent trainings, where, as Chapter 8 noted, the ecosystem is young and your questions must do the work that established credential structures do elsewhere.

Read the layers together and a rule of thumb emerges for trauma work: license first, specialty depth second, and for complex histories, evidence of consultation or supervision in that specialty third. A weekend course is exposure. Certification with consultation hours is depth. Depth is what you want holding the pointer.

Twelve Questions Worth Asking

Most good practitioners offer a brief consultation call, and the ones who do not offer one will usually answer questions by message. Here is the interview, and every question has a purpose you now understand from earlier chapters.

1. What is your core license, and where can I verify it?

2. What training have you completed in this specific method, and when?

3. Do you have ongoing consultation or supervision in it?

4. How much of your practice is trauma work, and with histories like mine?

5. How do you decide whether this method fits a particular person?

6. What does your preparation phase look like before any processing?

7. How do you keep sessions inside a client's window of tolerance?

8. How do you work with dissociation if it shows up?

9. What would make you adjust the approach or refer me elsewhere?

10. What is your experience delivering this by telehealth, if relevant?

11. What are your fees, session length, and cancellation terms?

12. What should I expect between sessions, and how do you handle a rough week?

Good answers are specific, calm, and unhurried, like the second call Carwen made. The best answers include the phrase it depends followed by what it depends on, because honest trauma work is conditional, and practitioners who know their method's edges will tell you about them without being cornered.

Red Flags in Plain Sight

Some warnings are visible from the first contact, and you should trust them. Guarantees of results, in any wording, misdescribe how this field works. Pressure to begin processing immediately, or dismissal of preparation as unnecessary for someone like you, contradicts the safety architecture every chapter of this book has described. Vagueness about training that survives a direct question is an answer in itself. So is any response to your framework page that treats your informed participation as an obstacle. And a practitioner offering a powerful specialty method without a verifiable foundation license is the one flag that ends the conversation regardless of everything else.

One flag is subtler and worth naming because good people miss it: the practitioner whose answer to every history is the single method they sell. You have spent nine chapters learning that legitimate therapies have centers and edges. Someone who has spent a career learning one method and found no edges has not been looking, and Meeka's first phone call in the last chapter failed on exactly this point.

Money, Time, and Screens

Practicalities, labeled as the estimates they are. Session fees vary so widely by country and region that any number printed here would mislead someone; what generalizes is the structure. Expect intake and preparation sessions before processing in any method. Expect single-incident work to be measured in a couple of months and complex work in seasons, as earlier chapters detailed. Ask insurers and public systems specifically about EMDR by name, since its guideline status is the lever, and ask any practitioner about sliding scales, because many quietly offer them. Telehealth is a legitimate route in all three methods, with the usual conditions: privacy on your end, a plan for grounding if a session runs hard, and a practitioner experienced in remote delivery, question ten on your list.

> **Action Challenge:** *A conversation task and then the behavior task this chapter was built for. First, rehearse the twelve questions aloud once, alone or with someone you trust, until asking them feels like diligence rather than rudeness, because it is diligence. Then, within two weeks, book one consultation call with a practitioner of your first-ranked method and run the interview. Not a commitment. A call. The gap between readers who heal and readers who research indefinitely is usually one phone call wide.*

The Call You Will Make

Verify the license, measure the depth, ask the twelve questions, and honor the flags, and the Practitioner Premium starts paying you instead of costing you. Somewhere reachable there is a version of Carwen's second call waiting for you, a person with specific training, honest edges, and an unhurried answer about safety. When you find them, the choosing is done and the work begins, and the final chapter of this book is about exactly that: the first six sessions, the doubts that visit them, and how to tell ordinary difficulty from a wrong turn.

Chapter 12: The First Six Sessions

Jump forward six weeks. The choosing is behind you, the consultation call went well, and you are three or four sessions into the therapy your grid ranked first. And something this book must tell you now, before you live it, is what those weeks are likely to contain: a good start, then a session that leaves you stirred and doubtful, then a week when the old symptoms visit loudly, and then, precisely on schedule, the thought that you chose wrong. Nearly everyone meets that thought. What separates outcomes is not whether it arrives but what you do when it does, and doing it well requires a principle set in advance, while you are calm, which is now.

I call it the Six Session Review: commit at the start to a fixed review point around the sixth session, with success markers written in advance, and until that point, treat doubt as data to record rather than a decision to act on. The principle works because early trauma treatment is genuinely noisy. Material is being contacted that was avoided for years, and a temporary stirring of sleep, dreams, emotion, and memory is documented across methods and expected by every competent practitioner. Deciding inside the noise means deciding on the noise. The review point moves the decision to a place with better light.

What Early Progress Actually Looks Like

Recalibrate your expectations away from the movies. Early progress in trauma therapy rarely announces itself as peace. It looks like Bindi's stubborn rating finally sliding, weeks in. It looks like Alora's clinic response softening while one trigger stayed loud. It looks like noticing, as Zowie did, an unguarded moment that would previously have been braced. Sometimes it even looks like feeling more for a while, because numbness lifting is progress wearing its most confusing costume. What you are watching for in the first six sessions is not resolution but movement: any change in the frequency, intensity, duration, or aftermath of your difficulty, and any growth in your sense of safety with the practitioner.

That last item is not soft garnish. The working alliance, your sense of being understood, respected, and safe with this person, is one of the most reliable early signals in all of psychotherapy research, across every method (Flückiger et al., 2018). If the technique is wobbling but the alliance is strong, you likely have a pacing problem, which is fixable. If the technique seems fine but you feel unseen or unsafe, you have a bigger problem than technique, whatever the method's trial results say.

Discomfort or Poor Fit

Here is the discernment this chapter exists to teach, in one table you can return to when the doubt arrives.

Signal	Ordinary difficulty	Poor fit or poor delivery
Hard sessions	Stirred, settles within days	Flooded, worse for a week or more
Between sessions	Noisy but functional	Escalating, destabilized
Window of tolerance	Stretched, not shattered	Repeatedly thrown outside it
Practitioner response	Adjusts pacing when told	Dismisses, pushes through
Direction	Something, anything, is moving by review	Nothing has moved at all
Alliance	Growing trust despite hard content	Growing dread of the sessions

The left column is the price of admission described honestly throughout this book. The right column is a pattern, and one entry alone rarely proves it, which is why the review point matters: patterns show themselves across six sessions in a way no single bad Tuesday can.

Say It Before You Leave

The single most underused move in all of therapy is the sentence spoken to the practitioner before it is spoken to a search engine. This is feeling like too much too fast. I left the last two sessions more flooded than I can settle. I keep disappearing in the middle and I am not sure you can tell. Competent practitioners in every method have adjustments waiting behind exactly these sentences, shorter sets, longer grounding, a return to preparation, a change of target, and the difference between a rescue and a rupture is often just whether the sentence got said. Say it in the room. If saying it is impossible, say it in a message before the next session. A practitioner who receives it well has just shown you the working alliance in action. One who receives it badly has completed your review early.

Switching Without Starting Over

Sometimes the review point arrives and the honest reading is poor fit. Hear this clearly: switching is a maneuver, not a defeat, and nothing you built transfers at zero. Your history is mapped. Your stabilization skills are trained. Your self-knowledge, the window tally, the edge locations, the whole notebook, moves with you, and your framework already holds a ranked second name for precisely this moment. When you switch, tell the new practitioner the full story of the stall, because Chapter 10 taught you that stall patterns are diagnostic gold, and a good clinician will design around them from session one.

Luan's year shows the maneuver done well, including its costs. Brainspotting was his grid's first rank, and four months of it moved real ground before progress flattened in a way the review framework made undeniable. Rather than grinding on loyalty, he and his practitioner talked it through openly, and she referred him onward herself, to a DBR-trained colleague, with a summary that spared him starting from nothing. The transition still cost him: a setback month while trust rebuilt, and a stretch of doubt he describes as louder than anything in the therapy itself. The second method reached the layer the first had circled. He ended the year substantially better and not finished, holding both therapies in genuine respect, and his one regret is the extra months he spent before the first switch because switching felt like failing.

Sequences and Combinations

Luan's path was not an anomaly, and this book ends its comparison by softening its own categories. Real healing careers are often sequences: stabilization in one modality, processing in another, grief work or behavioral change in a third, as Zowie's and Orson's stories already showed. Many practitioners are trained across the family tree from Chapter 2 and will themselves blend, following EMDR's structure into a Brainspotting hold, or preparing DBR-style bodywork inside a broader therapy. Comparative research keeps suggesting that legitimate trauma treatments share more effectiveness than their brands imply, which means a sequence is not indecision, it is coverage (Watkins et al., 2018). Your ranked list was never a tournament bracket. It is an itinerary, and some readers will use more than one line of it.

Keeping Score Honestly

The review needs data, so keep some, lightly. Once a week, the same day each week, write three numbers from zero to ten: how loud the main difficulty was this week, how functional you were around it, and how safe you feel in the therapy. Add one sentence of anything notable. Two minutes, no essays. At the sixth-session review, read the sequence aloud to yourself, place it against the table above, and against the success markers you set at the start. Then decide: continue, adjust, or activate the next name. Whatever you choose will be the most informed treatment decision most people ever get to make.

> **Action Challenge:** *Two tasks that complete this book's work. The writing task: tonight, before the first session if possible, write your three success markers, what movement would look like by session six in symptoms, in function, and in the alliance, and set the review date in your calendar by name. The behavior task: begin the weekly three-number score this week, whether or not therapy has started, so your baseline exists before the noise does.*

Keeping Your Own Score

Expect the doubt, schedule the review, speak the sentence before you leave, switch as a maneuver when the pattern is real, and let sequences count as strategy. That is the whole discipline of the first six sessions, and it converts the choice you made in Chapter 10 from a bet into a process with feedback. One short chapter remains, and it is not instruction. It is the view from the end of the map, and the beginning of the part no book can walk for you.

Conclusion

Morag, from the first page of this book, typed her question into a search bar at night: why is therapy not working for me. Thirteen chapters later, you hold the answer this book set out to give her. Therapy was not failing her, and she was not failing therapy. An upper-floor method had been assigned a basement problem, for years, and nobody had shown her the map of the building.

You now hold that map in unusual detail. You know why insight alone could not settle a body that stores trauma below language, and you know the family of therapies built for the descent: the structured, well-evidenced staircase of EMDR, the quiet doorway of Brainspotting, and the slow subbasement work of Deep Brain Reorienting. You have seen each room's best case and its honest edges, watched one man carry one wound through all three, and drawn the nine lines that truly divide them. More importantly, you have gathered evidence about the one subject no trial ever studied: your own nervous system, its window, its patterns, its address book, its vote.

And you have, if you did the work, a page this book could not have printed: a completed grid, a ranked list with reasons, twelve questions rehearsed, success markers drafted, and a review date waiting for a calendar. That page is the whole difference between reading about healing and beginning it.

Fit Before Fault, one last time, because it is the sentence to keep when the rest of this book fades. When a committed person and a legitimate method fail to help each other, examine the match before assigning blame. It reinterprets your past attempts as data. It disciplines your next choice. And it keeps you humane with yourself on the hard weeks ahead, when the old thought visits and calls the struggle a verdict. It is not a verdict. It is engineering, and you are now the best-informed engineer your healing has ever had.

Hold the map lightly as the territory changes. DBR's evidence file will thicken, one direction or another. New adaptations will reach the older methods. Your yearly afternoon of homework from Chapter 8 will keep the picture current, and the questions you learned to ask will outlast every snapshot in these pages.

Two final words, both of them practical. First: none of this replaces the professionals. The framework makes you an informed chooser; the choosing still finishes in conversation with a qualified clinician, and the healing happens in a relationship with one. If any part of your history involves risk to your safety, that conversation comes first, before any of this book's machinery. Second, the action that remains, the only one left unassigned: make the call. Not the perfect call after the final round of research. The consultation call, this week, with the first name on your page, twelve questions in hand.

Begin

Somewhere behind you is the night you typed the question. Somewhere ahead of you is an unguarded moment, a door that slams and a body that simply notices, the way Zowie caught herself unbraced, the way Phaedon stood under the scaffold and thought about lunch. Between those two points there is no mystery left, only a sequence you now know how to run: match, verify, ask, begin, review. The map is finished. The territory is yours. Begin.

References

American Psychological Association. (2017). Clinical practice guideline for the treatment of posttraumatic stress disorder (PTSD) in adults. American Psychological Association.

Bisson, J. I., Roberts, N. P., Andrew, M., Cooper, R., & Lewis, C. (2013). Psychological therapies for chronic post-traumatic stress disorder (PTSD) in adults. Cochrane Database of Systematic Reviews, 2013(12), Article CD003388. https://doi.org/10.1002/14651858.CD003388.pub4

Corrigan, F. M., & Christie-Sands, J. (2020). An innate brainstem self-other system involving orienting, affective responding, and polyvalent relational seeking: Some clinical implications for a Deep Brain Reorienting trauma psychotherapy approach. Medical Hypotheses, 136, Article 109502. https://doi.org/10.1016/j.mehy.2019.109502

Corrigan, F. M., & Grand, D. (2013). Brainspotting: Recruiting the midbrain for accessing and healing sensorimotor memories of traumatic activation. Medical Hypotheses, 80(6), 759-766. https://doi.org/10.1016/j.mehy.2013.03.005

Corrigan, F. M., Grand, D., & Raju, R. (2015). Brainspotting: Sustained attention, spinothalamic tracts, thalamocortical processing, and the healing of adaptive orientation truncated by traumatic experience. Medical Hypotheses, 84(4), 384-394. https://doi.org/10.1016/j.mehy.2015.01.028

Corrigan, F. M., Young, H., & Christie-Sands, J. (2025). Deep brain reorienting: Understanding the neuroscience of trauma, attachment wounding, and DBR psychotherapy. Routledge.

D'Antoni, F., Matiz, A., Fabbro, F., & Crescentini, C. (2022). Psychotherapeutic techniques for distressing memories: A comparative study between EMDR, brainspotting, and body scan meditation. International Journal of Environmental

Research and Public Health, 19(3), Article 1142. https://doi.org/10.3390/ijerph19031142

Ecker, B., Ticic, R., & Hulley, L. (2012). Unlocking the emotional brain: Eliminating symptoms at their roots using memory reconsolidation. Routledge.

Flückiger, C., Del Re, A. C., Wampold, B. E., & Horvath, A. O. (2018). The alliance in adult psychotherapy: A meta-analytic synthesis. Psychotherapy, 55(4), 316-340. https://doi.org/10.1037/pst0000172

Gonzalez-Vazquez, A. I., Rodriguez-Lago, L., Seoane-Pillado, M. T., Fernandez, I., Garcia-Guerrero, F., & Santed-German, M. A. (2018). The progressive approach to EMDR group therapy for complex trauma and dissociation: A case-control study. Frontiers in Psychology, 8, Article 2377. https://doi.org/10.3389/fpsyg.2017.02377

Grand, D. (2013). Brainspotting: The revolutionary new therapy for rapid and effective change. Sounds True.

Herman, J. L. (1992). Trauma and recovery. Basic Books.

Hildebrand, A., Grand, D., & Stemmler, M. (2017). Brainspotting: The efficacy of a new therapy approach for the treatment of posttraumatic stress disorder in comparison to eye movement desensitization and reprocessing. Mediterranean Journal of Clinical Psychology, 5(1), 1-17. https://doi.org/10.6092/2282-1619/2017.5.1376

Kearney, B. E., Corrigan, F. M., Frewen, P. A., Nevill, S., Harricharan, S., Andrews, K., Jetly, R., McKinnon, M. C., & Lanius, R. A. (2023). A randomized controlled trial of Deep Brain Reorienting: A neuroscientifically guided treatment for post-traumatic stress disorder. European Journal of Psychotraumatology, 14(2), Article 2240691. https://doi.org/10.1080/20008066.2023.2240691

Kearney, B. E., & Lanius, R. A. (2022). The brain-body disconnect: A somatic sensory basis for trauma-related disorders. Frontiers in Neuroscience, 16, Article 1015749. https://doi.org/10.3389/fnins.2022.1015749

Lanius, R. A., Vermetten, E., Loewenstein, R. J., Brand, B., Schmahl, C., Bremner, J. D., & Spiegel, D. (2010). Emotion modulation in PTSD: Clinical and neurobiological evidence for a dissociative subtype. American Journal of Psychiatry, 167(6), 640-647. https://doi.org/10.1176/appi.ajp.2009.09081168

LeDoux, J. (1996). The emotional brain: The mysterious underpinnings of emotional life. Simon & Schuster.

Levine, P. A. (1997). Waking the tiger: Healing trauma. North Atlantic Books.

Lewis, C., Roberts, N. P., Andrew, M., Starling, E., & Bisson, J. I. (2020). Psychological therapies for post-traumatic stress disorder in adults: Systematic review and meta-analysis. European Journal of Psychotraumatology, 11(1), Article 1729633. https://doi.org/10.1080/20008198.2020.1729633

Lewis, C., Roberts, N. P., Gibson, S., & Bisson, J. I. (2020). Dropout from psychological therapies for post-traumatic stress disorder (PTSD) in adults: Systematic review and meta-analysis. European Journal of Psychotraumatology, 11(1), Article 1709709. https://doi.org/10.1080/20008198.2019.1709709

Matthijssen, S. J. M. A., Brouwers, T., van Roozendaal, C., Vuister, T., & de Jongh, A. (2021). The effect of EMDR versus EMDR 2.0 on emotionality and vividness of aversive memories in a non-clinical sample. European Journal of Psychotraumatology, 12(1), Article 1956793. https://doi.org/10.1080/20008198.2021.1956793

National Institute for Health and Care Excellence. (2018). Post-traumatic stress disorder (NICE Guideline NG116). National Institute for Health and Care Excellence.

Ogden, P., Minton, K., & Pain, C. (2006). Trauma and the body: A sensorimotor approach to psychotherapy. W. W. Norton.

Porges, S. W. (2011). The polyvagal theory: Neurophysiological foundations of emotions, attachment, communication, and self-regulation. W. W. Norton.

Schottenbauer, M. A., Glass, C. R., Arnkoff, D. B., Tendick, V., & Gray, S. H. (2008). Nonresponse and dropout rates in outcome studies on PTSD: Review and methodological considerations. Psychiatry, 71(2), 134-168. https://doi.org/10.1521/psyc.2008.71.2.134

Shapiro, F. (2012). Getting past your past: Take control of your life with self-help techniques from EMDR therapy. Rodale.

Shapiro, F. (2018). Eye movement desensitization and reprocessing (EMDR) therapy: Basic principles, protocols, and procedures (3rd ed.). Guilford Press.

Siegel, D. J. (1999). The developing mind: How relationships and the brain interact to shape who we are. Guilford Press.

Stickgold, R. (2002). EMDR: A putative neurobiological mechanism of action. Journal of Clinical Psychology, 58(1), 61-75. https://doi.org/10.1002/jclp.1129

van den Hout, M. A., & Engelhard, I. M. (2012). How does EMDR work? Journal of Experimental Psychopathology, 3(5), 724-738. https://doi.org/10.5127/jep.028212

van der Kolk, B. A. (2014). The body keeps the score: Brain, mind, and body in the healing of trauma. Viking.

Wampold, B. E. (2015). How important are the common factors in psychotherapy? An update. World Psychiatry, 14(3), 270-277. https://doi.org/10.1002/wps.20238

Watkins, L. E., Sprang, K. R., & Rothbaum, B. O. (2018). Treating PTSD: A review of evidence-based psychotherapy interventions. Frontiers in Behavioral Neuroscience, 12, Article 258. https://doi.org/10.3389/fnbeh.2018.00258

World Health Organization. (2013). Guidelines for the management of conditions specifically related to stress. World Health Organization.

www.ingramcontent.com/pod-product-compliance
Lightning Source LLC
LaVergne TN
LVHW022313200926
848481LV00004B/1329